LIVING

With

MYASTHENIA GRAVIS

By

Dr. Barbara Smith

Copyright no part of this book should be written copied or sold without Authors permission

Table Of Contents

Introduction

As a practicing physician specializing in neurology, my journey with Myasthenia Gravis (MG) began not just within the walls of my clinic but through the stories and challenges faced by my patients. Witnessing the resilience and struggles of individuals grappling with MG has been a humbling and enlightening experience, one that sparked the impetus to pen this comprehensive guide, "Living Strong with Myasthenia Gravis."

In my clinical practice, I've encountered the complexities of this condition firsthand, witnessing its impact not only on the physical health but also on the emotional and social well-being of those affected. My patients' fortitude in facing the uncertainties and hurdles posed by MG has inspired me to delve deeper into understanding this autoimmune neuromuscular disorder and to compile a resource that navigates its multifaceted dimensions.

This book is a culmination of my dedication to providing comprehensive care to individuals living with MG. It aspires to be a guiding light, offering insights, practical strategies, and a roadmap for both patients and their caregivers as they navigate the challenges posed by this condition.

Within these pages, I aim to combine medical knowledge with practical advice, empowering readers with the tools to manage symptoms, comprehend treatment options, and lead fulfilling lives despite the hurdles posed by MG. Through this book, I hope to bridge the gap between medical expertise and the everyday experiences of those living with MG, offering not only information but also empathy, encouragement, and hope.

May this book serve as a companion, providing guidance, support, and reassurance to all individuals impacted by Myasthenia Gravis, fostering a sense of resilience and strength in the face of adversity.

Chapter 1

Introduction to Myasthenia Gravis

Defining Myasthenia Gravis (MG)

Myasthenia Gravis (MG) stands as an enigmatic but significant condition within the spectrum of autoimmune disorders affecting the neuromuscular junction. The name itself, derived from the Greek words "myasthenia" (muscle weakness) and "gravis" (serious), accurately encapsulates the primary hallmark of this ailment: muscle weakness of variable severity.

At its core, MG is characterized by the body's own immune system mistakenly attacking the receptors responsible for transmitting nerve signals to muscles. This disruptive process impedes the normal communication between nerves and muscles, leading to the characteristic muscle weakness and fatigue that define the condition.

Understanding the Neuromuscular Junction

To comprehend the nuances of Myasthenia Gravis, it's imperative to grasp the workings of the neuromuscular junction, a critical point of connection between nerve cells and muscle fibers. This intricate setup is where nerve impulses are transmitted to muscles, triggering muscle contractions essential for movement.

Within this junction, acetylcholine, a neurotransmitter, plays a pivotal role. Nerve cells release acetylcholine, which then binds to specific receptors on muscle cells, initiating muscle contractions. In Myasthenia Gravis, the immune system produces antibodies that target and attack these acetylcholine receptors, impeding their function. Consequently, the transmission of nerve signals to muscles becomes disrupted, leading to muscle weakness and fatigue, particularly during repetitive or sustained movements.

The Variability of Myasthenia Gravis

One of the intriguing and challenging aspects of MG lies in its variability. Its symptoms can range from mild to severe, and they often fluctuate over time. Some individuals might experience primarily ocular symptoms, such as drooping eyelids (ptosis) or double vision (diplopia), while others might encounter more generalized muscle weakness affecting various parts of the body, including limbs, neck, and respiratory muscles.

The onset of MG can occur at any age, but it's more commonly diagnosed in women under 40 and men over 60. The unpredictable nature of symptom manifestation and progression poses unique challenges, making MG a condition that requires ongoing management and tailored treatment approaches.

Brief History and Discovery

The story of Myasthenia Gravis is woven into the annals of medical history, marked by a journey of discovery, recognition, and continuous advancements in understanding this intriguing condition.

The roots of Myasthenia Gravis trace back to the late 19th century when French neurologist Jean-Martin Charcot and his contemporaries laid the groundwork for unraveling the complexities of neuromuscular diseases. However, it wasn't until the turn of the 20th century that the distinctive characteristics of MG began to emerge from the medical milieu.

In 1895, British physician Sir William Osler identified and described a series of cases marked by muscle weakness and fatigability. This collection of symptoms, later recognized as Myasthenia Gravis, piqued the interest of physicians and researchers alike. The term "myasthenia gravis" was coined in 1900 by German neurologist Wilhelm Erb, who aptly described the condition's hallmark features of severe muscle weakness.

The pivotal moment in the recognition of MG came in 1934 when neurologists Mary Walker and Lord Russell Brain discovered a link between muscle weakness and abnormalities at the neuromuscular junction. Their groundbreaking work laid the foundation for understanding the role of acetylcholine receptors and the immune system's involvement in the pathology of MG.

Advancements in medical technology and diagnostic techniques in the latter half of the 20th century further propelled the understanding of MG. The introduction of electromyography (EMG), the development of specific antibody tests targeting acetylcholine receptors, and imaging modalities contributed significantly to accurate diagnosis and delineation of various subtypes of MG.

The subsequent decades witnessed a surge in research endeavors, leading to the identification of additional antibodies involved in MG, unveiling novel treatment approaches, and paving the way for clinical trials exploring innovative therapies.

Today, the historical journey of Myasthenia Gravis serves as a testament to the collaborative efforts of healthcare professionals, researchers, and patients themselves. It signifies not only the strides made in unraveling the mysteries of this condition but also the promise of continued advancements aimed at improving the lives of individuals affected by MG.

In the subsequent sections of this book, we will delve deeper into the contemporary understanding of MG, its pathophysiology, diagnosis, treatment options, and the holistic management strategies that form the cornerstone of living well with this condition.

How MG Affects the Neuromuscular System

Myasthenia Gravis (MG) manifests its effects at the intricate junction where nerve signals meet muscle responsiveness - the neuromuscular junction. This convergence point is crucial for the transmission of nerve impulses that prompt muscle contractions, enabling movements essential for daily activities.

In MG, the body's immune system, typically as a result of autoimmunity, produces antibodies that target specific components within the neuromuscular junction. Primarily, these antibodies bind to the acetylcholine receptors present on the surface of muscle cells.

Acetylcholine receptors play a pivotal role in transmitting nerve signals to muscles. When acetylcholine, a neurotransmitter, is released from nerve endings, it binds to these receptors, initiating a cascade of events that result in muscle contraction. However, in individuals with MG, the presence of antibodies obstructs or even destroys these receptors, disrupting the normal signal transmission process.

As a consequence, the efficiency of communication between nerves and muscles diminishes significantly. With fewer functional receptors available to receive and process nerve signals, the muscles receive inadequate stimulation, leading to weakness and fatigue.

The impact of MG on the neuromuscular system isn't uniform; it exhibits variability in its effects. Depending on the extent of receptor impairment, the severity and distribution of muscle weakness can differ widely among individuals. Some may experience isolated weakness in specific muscles, such as those controlling eye movements, resulting in drooping eyelids (ptosis) or double vision (diplopia). Others may encounter more generalized muscle weakness, affecting limbs, facial muscles, swallowing, and even respiratory muscles.

Moreover, the symptoms of MG often worsen with prolonged or repetitive use of affected muscles, a phenomenon referred to as "fatigue." This fatigue is a hallmark feature of the condition and can significantly impact an individual's ability to perform tasks requiring sustained muscle use.

Chapter 2: Symptoms and

Diagnosis

Common Symptoms of Myasthenia

Gravis

Myasthenia Gravis (MG) is a complex condition that often presents with a spectrum of symptoms affecting various muscle groups. The symptoms can vary widely among individuals and may fluctuate in severity over time. Recognizing these hallmark signs is crucial for an accurate diagnosis and prompt initiation of appropriate management strategies.

1. Muscle Weakness: The most prevalent and defining symptom of MG is muscle weakness, which tends to

worsen with repeated or sustained use of affected muscles. This weakness often improves with rest. Common areas affected include the eyes, causing drooping eyelids (ptosis) and double vision (diplopia). Other muscles, such as those in the limbs, face, neck, and throat, can also be impacted, leading to difficulty in speaking, chewing, swallowing, or lifting objects.

2. Fatigue: Muscle fatigue is a distinctive feature of MG. Patients often report increased weakness or loss of muscle function after exertion or prolonged activity. This fatigue can significantly impact daily activities and may require periods of rest to regain muscle strength.

3. Respiratory Complications: In severe cases or during MG exacerbations, respiratory muscles can be affected, leading to breathing difficulties. Shortness of breath, especially during physical exertion or at night, could be indicative of respiratory muscle weakness, necessitating immediate medical attention.

4. Ocular Symptoms: About two-thirds of individuals with MG initially experience symptoms localized to the eyes. These may include drooping of one or both eyelids (ptosis) and double vision (diplopia). Ocular

symptoms in MG often result from weakness in the muscles that control eye movements.

5. Swallowing and Speech Difficulties: Weakness in the muscles involved in swallowing and speaking can lead to difficulties in swallowing (dysphagia) and changes in speech, such as slurred speech or a nasal tone.

6. Facial Muscle Weakness: Some individuals may exhibit weakness in facial muscles, resulting in a lack of facial expression or difficulty in facial movements like smiling or frowning.

Recognizing these common symptoms and their variability is fundamental in the diagnostic process for Myasthenia Gravis. However, it's essential to note that symptoms can differ significantly among individuals, and not all affected individuals experience the same combination or severity of symptoms. Seeking medical evaluation upon the onset of these symptoms is crucial for accurate diagnosis and timely intervention.

Challenges in Diagnosing Myasthenia Gravis

Diagnosing Myasthenia Gravis (MG) can present several challenges owing to the variability and mimicry of its symptoms, often resembling other neuromuscular or systemic conditions. This diagnostic complexity can result in delays or difficulties in accurately identifying MG in its early stages.

1. Symptom Variability: The spectrum of symptoms associated with MG can vary widely among individuals. Additionally, these symptoms may fluctuate in intensity over time or in response to various factors, making it challenging to establish a definitive pattern for diagnosis.

2. Overlapping Symptoms: The manifestations of MG, particularly muscle weakness and fatigue, may resemble symptoms of other neuromuscular or autoimmune disorders. This overlap often necessitates a thorough differential diagnosis to distinguish MG from conditions such as Lambert-Eaton myasthenic

syndrome (LEMS), multiple sclerosis, chronic fatigue syndrome, or certain muscular dystrophies.

3. Ocular Predominance and Progression: For some individuals, MG symptoms initially manifest predominantly in the eyes (ocular MG) before progressing to more generalized muscle weakness. However, this transition might not always occur linearly, further complicating the diagnostic process.

4. Diagnostic Tests Interpretation: While specific tests aid in the diagnosis of MG, such as the edrophonium test, repetitive nerve stimulation, single-fiber electromyography, and the detection of specific antibodies (e.g., anti-acetylcholine receptor antibodies), their interpretation can sometimes be challenging. False negatives or inconclusive results may occur, requiring further evaluation or additional testing for confirmation.

5. Coexistence with Other Conditions: MG can coexist with other autoimmune disorders, adding complexity to the diagnostic process. The presence of concurrent autoimmune conditions may complicate symptom interpretation and necessitate a comprehensive

evaluation to differentiate and manage these overlapping conditions effectively.

Diagnostic Tests and Procedures

Diagnosing Myasthenia Gravis (MG) involves a series of tests and procedures aimed at confirming the presence of the condition, differentiating it from other neuromuscular disorders, and determining its severity. A combination of clinical assessments, specialized tests, and imaging studies aids healthcare professionals in reaching an accurate diagnosis.

1. Clinical Evaluation: The diagnostic process often begins with a comprehensive medical history review and a detailed physical examination. Neurologists specialized in neuromuscular disorders focus on identifying specific signs indicative of MG, such as fluctuating muscle weakness, the presence of ptosis (drooping eyelids), diplopia (double vision), or difficulty in speaking or swallowing.

2. Neurological Examination: A thorough neurological assessment is crucial to evaluate muscle strength, reflexes, coordination, and sensory functions. Testing for muscle weakness and fatigability through

repetitive movements or specific maneuvers is fundamental in detecting characteristic signs of MG.

3. Antibody Testing: Detection of specific antibodies associated with MG aids in confirming the diagnosis. The presence of antibodies targeting components of the neuromuscular junction, such as acetylcholine receptors (AChR antibodies) or muscle-specific tyrosine kinase (MuSK antibodies), supports the diagnosis of MG.

4. Edrophonium Test: This test involves the administration of a short-acting medication called edrophonium chloride (Tensilon) to temporarily improve muscle strength in individuals with MG. Observation of a transient improvement in muscle weakness following the injection can provide additional evidence supporting the diagnosis.

5. Electrophysiological Studies: Specialized tests, including electromyography (EMG) and nerve conduction studies, help assess nerve and muscle function. Repetitive nerve stimulation and single-fiber EMG are particularly useful in detecting abnormal neuromuscular transmission, characteristic of MG.

6. Imaging Studies: In some cases, imaging modalities such as CT scans or MRI may be employed to assess the thymus gland, as abnormalities in this gland are associated with MG. Thymoma (a tumor of the thymus) is sometimes found in individuals with MG, and imaging helps evaluate its presence.

7. Pulmonary Function Tests: Evaluation of respiratory muscle function through pulmonary function tests or assessment of respiratory strength may be necessary to identify potential respiratory complications in severe cases of MG.

Collectively, these diagnostic tests and procedures serve as essential tools in confirming the diagnosis of Myasthenia Gravis, assessing its severity, and guiding the development of an appropriate treatment plan tailored to an individual's specific needs. Collaboration between healthcare providers specialized in neurology, neuromuscular diseases, and specialized testing facilities is crucial for an accurate diagnosis and effective management of MG.

Understanding Different Forms of MG:

Generalized, Ocular, and Other Variants

Myasthenia Gravis (MG) encompasses various clinical presentations, classified into distinct forms based on the distribution and severity of muscle weakness. Understanding these different variants is crucial, as they not only influence the pattern of symptoms but also aid in tailoring appropriate treatment strategies.

1. Generalized Myasthenia Gravis: This form of MG represents the most common presentation, characterized by muscle weakness affecting multiple muscle groups throughout the body. Individuals with generalized MG experience weakness in muscles controlling eye movements (resulting in ptosis and diplopia), facial muscles, limb muscles, respiratory muscles, and those involved in swallowing and speaking. Generalized MG can vary in severity from mild to severe and may require comprehensive management strategies.

2. Ocular Myasthenia Gravis: Ocular MG initially presents with symptoms localized to the eyes, involving weakness in the muscles that control eye movements. Ptosis (drooping eyelids) and diplopia (double vision) are typical manifestations of this variant. It's important to note that in some cases, ocular symptoms might progress to involve other muscle groups, transitioning into generalized MG over time. However, some individuals may continue to experience isolated ocular symptoms without progression.

3. Seronegative Myasthenia Gravis: In a subset of individuals with MG, specific antibodies associated with the condition, such as acetylcholine receptor antibodies (AChR) or muscle-specific tyrosine kinase antibodies (MuSK), may not be detectable through routine testing. This variant is referred to as seronegative MG. Despite the absence of detectable antibodies, clinical symptoms and response to treatment are indicative of MG.

4. Lambert-Eaton Myasthenic Syndrome (LEMS): LEMS shares some similarities with MG but is a distinct autoimmune disorder affecting neuromuscular

transmission. It involves autoantibodies targeting the calcium channels in nerve terminals, leading to impaired release of acetylcholine. LEMS often presents with muscle weakness, particularly affecting the legs, and is associated with certain underlying conditions, such as small-cell lung cancer.

Chapter 3: Causes and

Risk Factors

The Role of the Immune System in

Myasthenia Gravis (MG)

Myasthenia Gravis (MG) stands as a paradigm of autoimmune diseases, where the body's immune system, typically safeguarding against harmful invaders, mistakenly turns against its cells and tissues, leading to a cascade of events that underlie the pathology of this condition.

1. Autoimmunity and Antibody Production: In MG, the immune system generates antibodies that target components of the neuromuscular junction, specifically the acetylcholine receptors (AChR) or other proteins crucial for neuromuscular transmission, such as muscle-specific tyrosine kinase (MuSK). These antibodies disrupt the normal functioning of the acetylcholine receptors, impairing the transmission of nerve signals to muscles.

2. Disruption of Neuromuscular Communication: The antibodies produced in MG interfere with the binding of acetylcholine to its receptors on muscle cells. This interference hampers the transmission of nerve impulses, resulting in diminished muscle contractions and subsequent weakness, fatigue, and other associated symptoms.

3. Complement System Activation: Upon binding to the acetylcholine receptors, the antibodies in MG trigger the activation of the complement system—a part of the immune system responsible for immune responses against foreign invaders. This activation leads to the destruction or degradation of

acetylcholine receptors, further contributing to impaired neuromuscular transmission.

The precise trigger or initial cause of this immune system malfunction in MG remains a subject of ongoing research. Genetic predisposition, environmental factors, and potential triggers like viral infections are believed to contribute to the development of this autoimmune response in susceptible individuals. However, the exact interplay between these factors in initiating and perpetuating the immune system's attack on the neuromuscular junction in MG continues to be studied.

Potential Triggers and Risk Factors

Myasthenia Gravis (MG) is a multifactorial condition influenced by a combination of genetic predisposition, environmental factors, and potential triggers. While the exact cause of MG remains elusive, understanding the various risk factors and triggers associated with its development sheds light on its complex etiology.

1. Genetic Predisposition: Genetic factors play a role in predisposing individuals to MG. Certain genetic variations, although not deterministic, are believed to contribute to an increased susceptibility to autoimmune diseases, including MG. Human leukocyte antigen (HLA) genes, particularly the HLA-B8 and HLA-DR3 variants, have been associated with an elevated risk of developing MG in some populations. However, MG does not strictly follow a Mendelian inheritance pattern and likely involves multiple genetic factors.

2. Autoimmune and Immunological Factors: MG is primarily considered an autoimmune disorder,

indicating that the immune system malfunctions and mistakenly attacks the body's tissues. An imbalance or dysregulation within the immune system, involving T cells, B cells, and the production of autoantibodies against components of the neuromuscular junction (such as acetylcholine receptors or MuSK), contributes to the pathogenesis of MG.

3. Environmental Factors: Certain environmental triggers or exposures may influence the onset or exacerbation of MG in genetically predisposed individuals. Viral infections, such as Epstein-Barr virus (EBV), cytomegalovirus (CMV), or other respiratory infections, have been implicated as potential triggers that initiate or exacerbate MG in susceptible individuals. Additionally, factors like stress, pregnancy, hormonal changes, and certain medications have been proposed as potential triggers, although their precise role in the development of MG requires further investigation.

4. Thymus Abnormalities: The thymus gland, a key component of the immune system involved in the maturation of T cells, has been linked to MG. Abnormalities in the thymus, such as thymoma (a tumor of the thymus) or thymic hyperplasia (an

overgrowth of thymic tissue), are observed in a subset of individuals with MG. These thymic abnormalities are believed to contribute to the production of autoantibodies against the neuromuscular junction components.

Genetics and Predisposition to MG

Myasthenia Gravis (MG) involves a complex interplay between genetic predisposition and environmental factors, with genetics playing a significant role in determining an individual's susceptibility to this autoimmune disorder.

1. Human Leukocyte Antigen (HLA) Genes: Among the various genetic factors associated with MG, the involvement of certain human leukocyte antigen (HLA) genes has garnered considerable attention. HLA genes, which play a critical role in the immune system by presenting antigens to immune cells, exhibit variations that influence an individual's susceptibility to autoimmune diseases, including MG.

- HLA-B8 and HLA-DR3 Variants: These variants within the HLA complex have been identified in some populations as conferring an increased risk of developing MG. Studies have shown a higher prevalence of these variants in individuals diagnosed with MG compared to the general population. However, it's important to note that possessing these genetic variants does not guarantee the development of MG but rather increases the susceptibility to autoimmune conditions.

2. Non-HLA Genetic Factors: In addition to the HLA genes, research suggests the involvement of other non-HLA genetic factors in predisposing individuals to MG. Genome-wide association studies (GWAS) and genetic analyses have identified potential genetic variations outside the HLA region associated with an increased risk of MG. These genetic polymorphisms affect various components involved in immune regulation, including genes related to T cell function, B cell responses, and the production of autoantibodies targeting the neuromuscular junction.

3. Familial Clustering and Inheritance Patterns: While MG does not exhibit a straightforward pattern of inheritance, familial clustering has been observed, indicating a potential genetic component. Individuals with a family history of MG have a higher risk of developing the condition compared to the general population. However, the inheritance pattern appears to be multifactorial, involving the interaction of multiple genetic and environmental factors rather

than adhering strictly to Mendelian inheritance patterns.

4. Polygenic Nature of MG: Myasthenia Gravis is considered a polygenic disorder, meaning it involves multiple genetic variations across different genes, each contributing a modest effect to an individual's overall risk of developing the condition. This polygenic nature underscores the complexity of MG, making it challenging to pinpoint specific genetic determinants responsible for its onset.

While genetics play a significant role in predisposing individuals to MG, the development of the disorder results from a complex interplay between genetic susceptibility and environmental triggers. The identification of genetic markers associated with MG enhances our understanding of the underlying mechanisms and provides avenues for further research into personalized approaches for diagnosis, prognosis, and targeted therapeutic interventions tailored to an individual's genetic profile.

Chapter 4: Treatment

Options

Medications for Managing MG

Symptoms

Treating Myasthenia Gravis (MG) primarily aims at improving muscle strength, minimizing symptoms, and preventing disease exacerbations. Various medications play crucial roles in managing MG symptoms by modulating the immune system, enhancing neuromuscular transmission, or reducing the body's immune response against the neuromuscular junction components.

1. Acetylcholinesterase Inhibitors: Medications such as pyridostigmine (Mestinon) belong to this class of drugs, working by inhibiting the enzyme acetylcholinesterase. By blocking the breakdown of acetylcholine, these drugs increase the availability of acetylcholine at the neuromuscular junction, temporarily improving muscle strength and reducing symptoms of muscle weakness. Acetylcholinesterase inhibitors are commonly used to alleviate mild to moderate MG symptoms.

2. Corticosteroids: Prednisone and other corticosteroids are frequently prescribed in MG treatment to suppress the immune system's activity and reduce inflammation. These medications help control the autoimmune response that leads to the production of antibodies targeting the neuromuscular junction. Corticosteroids are particularly beneficial in managing generalized MG and preventing disease exacerbations, but their long-term use may be associated with side effects.

3. Immunomodulating Therapies: Other immunosuppressive agents, including azathioprine, mycophenolate mofetil, methotrexate, cyclosporine, and tacrolimus, are used in MG management. These medications target different aspects of the immune system, aiming to reduce the production of autoantibodies and dampen the immune response against the neuromuscular junction components. They are often employed as steroid-sparing agents or in combination with corticosteroids for long-term MG management.

4. Intravenous Immunoglobulin (IVIG): IVIG therapy involves the administration of high doses of immunoglobulins derived from pooled human blood plasma. IVIG modulates the immune system, temporarily suppressing the abnormal immune response in MG. It is used as a short-term intervention in severe MG exacerbations or as a maintenance therapy in individuals who do not tolerate other immunosuppressive treatments.

5. Plasma Exchange (Plasmapheresis): Plasma exchange involves removing the plasma containing harmful antibodies from the blood and replacing it with a substitute, such as albumin or donor plasma.

This procedure helps remove circulating autoantibodies and inflammatory mediators contributing to MG symptoms. Plasma exchange is often used as a short-term intervention to rapidly improve muscle strength in severe cases or as a bridge therapy while initiating long-term immunosuppressive treatments.

Thymectomy: Surgery for MG

Thymectomy, the surgical removal of the thymus gland, stands as a prominent therapeutic approach in the management of Myasthenia Gravis (MG), particularly in cases involving thymoma or when the thymus shows abnormal changes.

1. Rationale for Thymectomy: The rationale behind thymectomy stems from the association between the thymus gland and the development of MG. The thymus plays a pivotal role in the maturation of immune cells, and abnormalities within the thymus, such as the presence of thymoma (a tumor of the thymus) or thymic hyperplasia (an overgrowth of thymic tissue), have been observed in a subset of individuals with MG. Removal of the thymus aims to eliminate the potential source of abnormal immune responses and reduce the production of autoantibodies targeting the neuromuscular junction.

2. Surgical Procedure: Thymectomy can be performed via various approaches, including sternotomy (an

incision through the breastbone), minimally invasive techniques (such as video-assisted thoracoscopic surgery - VATS), or robotic-assisted surgery. The choice of approach depends on factors such as the patient's condition, the extent of thymic involvement, and the surgeon's expertise.

3. Efficacy of Thymectomy: Thymectomy has been shown to be beneficial, especially in specific subgroups of MG patients, including those under 60 years old with generalized MG, those with thymoma, or those with thymic hyperplasia. Studies have indicated that thymectomy, when performed early after MG diagnosis, can lead to improved clinical outcomes, increased likelihood of achieving remission, and reduced reliance on immunosuppressive medications.

4. Timing and Considerations: The optimal timing for thymectomy in MG remains a subject of debate. Some evidence suggests that early thymectomy, within the first few years of symptom onset, may result in better outcomes. However, its efficacy in older individuals or those with less thymic pathology is less established. Shared decision-making between patients and their healthcare providers is crucial in determining the

suitability and timing of thymectomy based on individual factors and preferences.

Thymectomy remains a valuable therapeutic option in the comprehensive management of MG, especially in selected patient populations. However, the decision to undergo thymectomy should be carefully weighed and discussed with a multidisciplinary team of specialists to assess its potential benefits and risks on a case-by-case basis.

Plasma Exchange and Intravenous

Immunoglobulin (IVIG) Therapy

Plasma exchange and Intravenous Immunoglobulin (IVIG) therapy serve as valuable treatment modalities, especially in severe cases, acute exacerbations, or as adjunctive therapies in individuals who do not respond adequately to other treatments.

1. Plasma Exchange (Plasmapheresis): Plasma exchange, also known as plasmapheresis, involves a procedure where blood is withdrawn from the patient, separated from the plasma containing harmful antibodies, and then reinfused with a substitute solution (such as albumin or donor plasma) to replace the removed plasma. This therapeutic intervention aims to remove circulating autoantibodies and inflammatory mediators contributing to MG symptoms. Plasma exchange is particularly beneficial in rapidly improving muscle strength in severe MG exacerbations, preoperative optimization before thymectomy, or as a temporary intervention while initiating long-term immunosuppressive treatments.

2. Intravenous Immunoglobulin (IVIG) Therapy: IVIG therapy involves administering high doses of immunoglobulins obtained from pooled human blood plasma through intravenous infusion. IVIG exerts its therapeutic effects by modulating the immune system, temporarily suppressing the abnormal immune response associated with MG. This treatment option is employed as a short-term intervention in severe MG exacerbations or as a maintenance therapy in individuals who do not tolerate other immunosuppressive treatments. IVIG has shown efficacy in improving muscle strength and reducing symptoms, especially in acute episodes of MG.

3. Mechanism of Action: Both plasma exchange and IVIG therapy work by modifying the immune system's function. Plasma exchange physically removes pathogenic antibodies and inflammatory mediators from the blood, whereas IVIG therapy delivers a pool of normal immunoglobulins, saturating Fc receptors on immune cells, interfering with the binding of autoantibodies, and modulating immune cell activities. These interventions result in a transient suppression of the abnormal immune response in MG, leading to symptomatic relief.

4. Considerations and Usage: Both plasma exchange and IVIG therapy are considered as short-term interventions rather than long-term solutions in MG management. They are typically utilized in acute exacerbations, preoperative optimization before thymectomy, or as a bridge therapy while initiating or adjusting long-term immunosuppressive treatments. The choice between plasma exchange and IVIG often depends on factors such as disease severity, patient response, availability, and specific clinical scenarios.

Plasma exchange and IVIG therapy serve as valuable therapeutic options in the armamentarium against Myasthenia Gravis, providing rapid relief and stabilization in acute situations. Their use in conjunction with other treatment modalities aims to optimize outcomes and improve the quality of life for individuals affected by this complex autoimmune condition.

Emerging Treatments and Clinical Trials

1. Complement Inhibitors: Emerging therapies targeting the complement system, such as eculizumab, ravulizumab, and zilucoplan, focus on inhibiting the complement cascade, which contributes to the destruction of acetylcholine receptors and exacerbates neuromuscular transmission impairment in MG. Clinical trials investigating complement inhibitors have shown promise in reducing disease severity, improving symptoms, and enhancing the quality of life for individuals with refractory MG.

2. B-cell Targeted Therapies: Biologic agents targeting B cells, including rituximab and ofatumumab, aim to deplete B cells involved in the production of autoantibodies targeting the neuromuscular junction in MG. By reducing the number of autoantibody-producing B cells, these therapies modulate the abnormal immune response. Clinical trials exploring the efficacy of B-cell targeted therapies have exhibited encouraging results in certain subsets of MG patients, especially those with treatment-resistant or refractory disease.

3. New Immunomodulatory Agents: Investigational immunomodulatory agents, such as rozanolixizumab and nipocalimab, focus on modulating immune cell function or inhibiting specific pathways involved in the immune response in MG. These agents show potential in altering the immune system's activity, suppressing the production of autoantibodies, and preserving neuromuscular function. Clinical trials assessing the safety and efficacy of these novel agents are ongoing, offering hope for more targeted and effective treatments.

4. Repurposed Drugs and Therapies: Exploration of repurposed drugs, such as fingolimod (used in multiple sclerosis) or idebenone (an antioxidant), showcases potential alternative treatment options for MG. These therapies, originally developed for other conditions, exhibit mechanisms of action that may confer benefits in modulating the immune response or enhancing neuromuscular transmission in MG. Clinical trials evaluating the repurposed drugs' safety and efficacy in MG management are underway.

5. Personalized Medicine Approaches: Advancements in understanding the genetic and immunological

profiles of individuals with MG pave the way for personalized treatment strategies. Tailoring treatments based on a patient's genetic, immunological, and clinical characteristics aims to optimize therapeutic outcomes and minimize adverse effects, fostering a more individualized approach in MG management.

Chapter 5: Living with Myasthenia Gravis: Daily Management

Coping Strategies for Fatigue and Muscle Weakness

Living with MG often involves navigating daily challenges related to muscle weakness and fatigue. Implementing effective coping strategies can significantly improve one's quality of life and help manage the impact of these symptoms. Here are several strategies to cope with fatigue and muscle weakness:

1. Prioritize Activities and Rest: Conserve energy by prioritizing essential tasks and scheduling them during times of the day when energy levels are higher. Balancing activities with adequate periods of rest throughout the day can prevent excessive fatigue and help manage muscle weakness.

2. Use Energy-Saving Techniques: Employ energy-saving techniques and adaptive strategies to minimize the strain on weakened muscles. For instance, use assistive devices or tools that reduce effort, optimize posture, and simplify tasks. Breaking tasks into smaller, manageable steps can also alleviate fatigue.

3. Plan and Organize Daily Activities: Organize tasks efficiently by planning in advance. Creating daily schedules or to-do lists helps distribute activities evenly throughout the day, preventing overexertion and fatigue accumulation.

4. Incorporate Regular Exercise: Engage in a tailored exercise program under the guidance of a healthcare professional or physical therapist. Specific exercises can help maintain muscle strength, improve endurance, and manage symptoms. However, exercises should be adjusted to individual capabilities and should account for periods of fatigue or weakness.

5. Manage Stress: Stress can exacerbate MG symptoms. Implement stress-reducing techniques such as meditation, deep breathing exercises, yoga, or mindfulness practices to help manage stress levels. Stress management techniques can aid in minimizing symptom flare-ups triggered by stress.

6. Balanced Nutrition: Maintain a well-balanced diet rich in nutrients, as nutrition plays a vital role in overall health and energy levels. Adequate hydration, along with a diet rich in fruits, vegetables, lean proteins, and whole grains, supports overall well-being and can help manage fatigue.

7. Seek Support: Establish a support network comprising healthcare professionals, family, friends, and support groups specializing in MG. Sharing

experiences, seeking advice, and receiving support from others facing similar challenges can provide valuable emotional support and practical tips for coping.

Balancing Physical Activity and Rest

Finding the right balance between physical activity and rest is crucial for individuals managing Myasthenia Gravis (MG). Striking this balance optimizes energy levels, minimizes symptom exacerbation, and preserves muscle function. Consider the following strategies to maintain this equilibrium:

1. Listen to Your Body: Pay close attention to your body's signals. Recognize signs of fatigue or muscle weakness, and take breaks when needed. Pushing through exhaustion may exacerbate symptoms and lead to prolonged recovery periods.

2. Pacing Activities: Adopt a pacing strategy that involves alternating periods of activity with periods of rest. Break tasks into manageable segments and intersperse rest periods to avoid overexertion. Avoiding prolonged periods of physical strain can help conserve energy and prevent fatigue.

3. Utilize Energy Conservation Techniques: Optimize energy use by incorporating energy-saving techniques

into daily activities. For instance, sit rather than stand while performing tasks, use supportive equipment or assistive devices to reduce muscle strain, and delegate tasks or ask for assistance when necessary.

4. Plan and Prioritize Activities: Plan activities wisely by scheduling demanding tasks during periods of higher energy levels. Prioritize tasks to focus on essential activities, allowing for adequate rest intervals between tasks to prevent fatigue accumulation.

5. Gradual Exercise: Engage in a tailored exercise program designed in consultation with a healthcare professional or physical therapist. Gradual, low-impact exercises can help maintain muscle strength and endurance without causing excessive fatigue. Begin with gentle exercises and gradually increase intensity or duration based on individual tolerance.

6. Adjust to Fluctuating Symptoms: Understand that MG symptoms can fluctuate. Be flexible in modifying activity levels based on daily variations in symptom severity. Adjustments in activity intensity or duration might be necessary on days when symptoms are more pronounced.

7. Practice Mindfulness: Incorporate mindfulness techniques into daily routines. Mindfulness exercises, such as deep breathing or meditation, can aid in managing stress and improving overall well-being. They also serve as relaxation tools to reduce muscle tension and fatigue.

Striking a balance between physical activity and rest is a dynamic process in MG management. It involves adapting to individual symptom variations, being mindful of personal limitations, and adopting strategies that promote optimal energy conservation. By fine-tuning activity levels and incorporating adequate rest, individuals with MG can better manage symptoms, optimize function, and enhance their overall quality of life.

Dietary Considerations and Nutrition

Tips

Maintaining a well-balanced diet and paying attention to nutritional intake are vital aspects of managing Myasthenia Gravis (MG). A healthy diet supports overall well-being, aids in managing symptoms, and helps optimize energy levels. Consider the following dietary considerations and nutrition tips:

1. Balanced Diet: Aim for a well-rounded diet rich in nutrients. Include a variety of foods from all food groups to ensure adequate intake of vitamins, minerals, proteins, carbohydrates, and healthy fats. A balanced diet provides essential nutrients crucial for maintaining optimal health and supporting muscle function.

2. Adequate Hydration: Stay well-hydrated by consuming sufficient fluids throughout the day. Dehydration can exacerbate symptoms of fatigue, so aim to drink water regularly. Proper hydration supports muscle function and overall body function.

3. Protein-Rich Foods: Incorporate lean protein sources such as poultry, fish, tofu, legumes, nuts, and seeds into your meals. Protein is essential for muscle repair and maintenance, aiding in preserving muscle strength.

4. Antioxidant-Rich Foods: Consume plenty of fruits and vegetables rich in antioxidants, such as berries, citrus fruits, leafy greens, carrots, and bell peppers. Antioxidants help combat oxidative stress, which can contribute to overall muscle health.

5. Balanced Meals Throughout the Day: Eat smaller, frequent meals throughout the day to maintain steady energy levels and prevent fluctuations in blood sugar levels. Avoid large, heavy meals that may induce fatigue.

6. Manageable Portion Sizes: Be mindful of portion sizes to prevent overeating, which can lead to discomfort and fatigue. Eating smaller, balanced portions can aid in digestion and prevent excessive strain on the body.

7. Consider Supplements if Necessary: Consult a healthcare professional to determine if specific supplements or vitamins, such as vitamin D, B-complex vitamins, or calcium, are necessary to supplement the diet. Nutritional supplements may be recommended based on individual needs and deficiencies.

8. Be Mindful of Medication Interactions: Some medications used in MG management may interact with certain foods or supplements. Discuss potential interactions or dietary restrictions with your healthcare provider to optimize medication efficacy and prevent adverse effects.

9. Seek Guidance from a Registered Dietitian: Consider seeking guidance from a registered dietitian or nutritionist specializing in MG or autoimmune conditions. They can provide personalized dietary advice, address nutritional concerns, and help create meal plans tailored to your specific needs.

Tips for Managing Stress and Promoting Emotional Well-being

Managing stress and maintaining emotional well-being are essential aspects of coping with Myasthenia Gravis (MG). The condition's fluctuating nature and its impact on daily life can be emotionally challenging. Incorporating strategies to manage stress and foster emotional wellness can significantly improve overall quality of life. Consider the following tips:

1. Stress Management Techniques: Explore various stress management techniques, such as deep breathing exercises, progressive muscle relaxation, mindfulness meditation, or yoga. These techniques help reduce stress levels and promote relaxation, easing both physical and emotional tension.

2. Establish Support Networks: Build a strong support system consisting of family, friends, healthcare professionals, and support groups specializing in MG. Connecting with others who understand the challenges of living with MG can provide valuable

emotional support, encouragement, and practical advice.

3. Open Communication: Maintain open communication with loved ones, caregivers, and healthcare providers about your feelings, concerns, and needs. Expressing emotions and discussing challenges openly can alleviate stress and foster understanding among those providing support.

4. Set Realistic Expectations: Be realistic about what you can accomplish and accept that MG symptoms may fluctuate. Avoid setting overly high expectations and be flexible in adapting to changing circumstances. Celebrate small achievements and milestones.

5. Engage in Enjoyable Activities: Participate in activities that bring joy and relaxation. Engaging in hobbies, creative pursuits, reading, listening to music, or spending time in nature can serve as therapeutic outlets and distract from MG-related stressors.

6. Maintain a Positive Outlook: Focus on maintaining a positive mindset and finding optimism in daily life. Cultivate gratitude by acknowledging and

appreciating the positives, however small they may seem.

7. Seek Professional Help: If feelings of anxiety, depression, or overwhelming stress persist, consider seeking support from mental health professionals, such as therapists, counselors, or psychologists. Professional guidance can assist in developing coping strategies and managing emotional challenges effectively.

8. Practice Self-care: Prioritize self-care by getting adequate sleep, maintaining a healthy diet, exercising regularly (within personal capabilities), and setting aside time for relaxation and rejuvenation. Taking care of yourself physically contributes to emotional resilience.

9. Educate Yourself: Knowledge is empowering. Learn more about MG through reputable sources, understand your condition, and engage in self-management strategies. Being informed can reduce uncertainty and empower you to take an active role in managing your health.

Chapter 6: Navigating

Relationships and Social

Life

Communicating with Family, Friends and

Colleagues about MG

Open and effective communication with family and friends is essential when dealing with Myasthenia Gravis (MG). Discussing MG with your loved ones can foster understanding, support, and collaboration in managing the condition. Here are some tips on communicating about MG:

1. Education and Information Sharing: Start by educating your family and friends about MG. Provide them with reliable resources or informational materials that explain the condition, its symptoms, potential challenges, and available treatments. Help them understand that MG is a chronic autoimmune disorder affecting neuromuscular function and that its symptoms may fluctuate.

2. Encourage Questions and Discussions: Encourage an open dialogue where your loved ones can ask questions, express their concerns, and seek clarification about MG. Allow them to voice their thoughts and emotions, creating a supportive environment for mutual understanding.

3. Share Personal Experiences: Share your personal experiences with MG, including how it affects your daily life, the symptoms you experience, and the impact it has on your physical and emotional well-being. Sharing specific examples can help your family and friends comprehend the challenges you face.

4. Be Honest and Realistic: Be honest about the limitations MG may impose on your activities, energy

levels, and overall functioning. Help your loved ones understand that while you strive to manage the condition, there might be times when adjustments or accommodations are necessary.

5. Express Your Needs: Clearly communicate your needs, whether it's for practical support, understanding during symptom exacerbations, or simply someone to listen. Articulate how your loved ones' support can positively impact your journey with MG.

6. Offer Practical Suggestions: Provide practical suggestions on how family and friends can support you, such as assisting with specific tasks during periods of fatigue, being flexible with plans when symptoms flare up, or offering emotional support through active listening.

7. Address Misconceptions: Address any misconceptions or myths surrounding MG to prevent misunderstandings. Correcting misinformation and providing accurate information about the condition can foster a more supportive and empathetic environment.

8. Patience and Understanding: Encourage patience and understanding among family and friends. MG's variable nature may be challenging to grasp initially, so allow time for them to comprehend and adjust to the impact of the condition on your life.

9. Appreciate Their Support: Express gratitude for the support and understanding your loved ones offer. Acknowledging their efforts can strengthen relationships and create a supportive network.

Chapter 7: Pregnancy,

Parenting, and MG

MG Considerations During Pregnancy

Pregnancy is a unique journey, and for women managing Myasthenia Gravis (MG), it requires careful planning and management. MG can present specific considerations during pregnancy. Here are key points to consider:

1. Preconception Planning: Before conceiving, consult with your healthcare provider, ideally a neurologist or a healthcare team experienced in managing MG. Discuss your plans for pregnancy, medications you're taking, and their potential effects on pregnancy and MG symptoms.

2. Medication Management: Review your current medication regimen with your healthcare provider. Some medications used to manage MG may need adjustments or alternative options during pregnancy to minimize potential risks to the fetus while ensuring adequate symptom control for the mother.

3. MG Symptom Monitoring: Pregnancy might affect MG symptoms. Some women experience improvements in symptoms during pregnancy, while others might see exacerbations. Regular monitoring by healthcare professionals is crucial to manage any changes in symptoms or disease activity.

4. Multidisciplinary Care: Collaborate with a multidisciplinary healthcare team, including obstetricians, neurologists, and potentially high-risk pregnancy specialists. Coordinated care ensures a comprehensive approach to managing both the pregnancy and MG.

5. Potential Risks: While most women with MG have successful pregnancies, there might be an increased risk of complications such as preterm birth, miscarriage, or exacerbation of MG symptoms. Discuss

these potential risks with your healthcare team to prepare and manage any unforeseen complications.

6. Delivery Planning: Develop a birth plan with your healthcare providers that considers your MG status. Discuss pain management options during labor, potential impact of anesthesia, and the need for monitoring MG symptoms during and after delivery.

7. Breastfeeding Considerations: Evaluate the compatibility of MG medications with breastfeeding. Some medications used to manage MG may pass into breast milk, potentially affecting the baby. Discuss breastfeeding options with your healthcare provider to make an informed decision.

8. Emotional Support: Pregnancy can be emotionally overwhelming, especially when managing a chronic condition like MG. Seek emotional support from healthcare providers, support groups, family, or counselors to navigate the emotional aspects of pregnancy and MG.

9. Postpartum Care: Prepare for postpartum care, as the early months after delivery might pose challenges in managing MG symptoms while caring for a

newborn. Ensure a support system in place to assist with daily tasks and caregiving responsibilities.

Support Networks for Families Affected

by MG

Living with Myasthenia Gravis (MG) impacts not only the individual but also their entire family. Accessing support networks and resources tailored to the needs of families affected by MG can be invaluable. Consider the following support options:

1. MG Support Groups: Join local or online MG support groups specifically catering to families. These groups provide a platform for sharing experiences, seeking advice, and connecting with others facing similar challenges. They offer emotional support, practical tips, and a sense of community.

2. Patient Advocacy Organizations: Numerous patient advocacy organizations and foundations focus on MG. These organizations offer resources, educational materials, and support services for individuals and families affected by MG. They often provide information about local support groups, educational events, and advocacy initiatives.

3. Healthcare Provider Networks: Establish a strong network of healthcare providers experienced in managing MG. Collaborate with neurologists, pediatricians (if parenting a child with MG), therapists, and other specialists to ensure comprehensive care and support for both the individual with MG and their family members.

4. Online Forums and Social Media: Explore online forums, blogs, and social media platforms dedicated to MG. These platforms serve as avenues for sharing experiences, asking questions, and accessing a wealth of information from a global community of individuals affected by MG.

5. Family Counseling or Therapy: Consider family counseling or therapy sessions to address the emotional impact of MG on family dynamics. Professional counseling can help family members better understand the challenges and foster healthy communication and support within the family unit.

6. Educational Resources: Access educational materials and reliable sources of information about MG tailored for families. Resources such as brochures, websites, or

publications provide valuable insights into understanding the condition, its management, and how it affects family life.

7. Peer Mentorship Programs: Some organizations offer peer mentorship programs where individuals or families new to MG can connect with seasoned mentors. Peer mentors provide guidance, emotional support, and practical advice based on their own experiences with MG.

8. Community Services and Respite Care: Investigate community services or respite care options available to provide temporary relief for caregivers or family members supporting an individual with MG. Respite care services offer a break for caregivers to recharge.

9. School and Educational Support: If a child in the family has MG, collaborate with the school or educational institution to create a supportive environment. Educate teachers, school staff, and classmates about MG to ensure understanding and accommodate the child's needs.

Living with Myasthenia Gravis

Chapter 8: Living a

Fulfilling Life with MG

Pursuing Hobbies and Interests

Living a fulfilling life with Myasthenia Gravis (MG) involves embracing hobbies and interests that bring joy, fulfillment, and a sense of purpose. Engaging in hobbies, despite the challenges posed by MG, can contribute significantly to one's overall well-being. Pursuing hobbies offers a way to explore passions, express creativity, and maintain a positive outlook despite the limitations imposed by the condition.

For individuals with MG, discovering hobbies that align with their energy levels and physical capabilities is crucial. Exploring low-energy activities such as painting, drawing, knitting, or reading can provide a creative outlet and a source of relaxation. These activities can be adapted to accommodate fluctuating energy levels, allowing individuals to engage at their own pace and convenience.

Adapting hobbies to suit personal abilities and limitations is essential. Considering alternative approaches or modifying activities allows individuals to continue pursuing interests while managing MG symptoms. Embracing hobbies that promote mental stimulation, such as puzzles, board games, or learning new skills online, can be fulfilling and enjoyable without requiring excessive physical exertion.

Moreover, exploring hobbies that offer opportunities for social interaction can enhance the overall experience. Participating in community groups, book clubs, or online forums related to shared interests creates connections and fosters a sense of belonging, despite the challenges posed by MG. These interactions not only provide support but also offer avenues for personal growth and social engagement.

Ultimately, the key to pursuing hobbies with MG lies in finding activities that bring joy, fulfillment, and a sense of accomplishment while respecting personal limitations. By embracing hobbies that align with individual capabilities and interests, individuals can enhance their quality of life, foster a positive mindset, and find moments of joy amid the challenges of living with MG.

Traveling with MG: Tips and Precautions

Traveling can be enriching, but for individuals managing Myasthenia Gravis (MG), it requires careful planning and considerations to ensure a smooth and enjoyable experience. Here are tips and precautions for traveling with MG:

- Plan Ahead: Research your destination and make necessary arrangements in advance. Identify healthcare facilities, pharmacies, and support services available at your destination. Carry sufficient medication and a copy of your medical records, including MG diagnosis and treatment details.

- Consult Your Healthcare Provider: Discuss your travel plans with your healthcare provider. Seek advice on adjusting medication schedules, managing symptoms during travel, and potential risks or precautions specific to your destination.

- Consider Travel Insurance: Obtain travel insurance that covers your medical needs, including MG-related emergencies or unexpected health issues. Understand the policy coverage, including pre-existing conditions.

- Pack Wisely: Pack essential medications, extra doses, and any necessary medical supplies in your carry-on luggage. Ensure you have adequate supplies for the duration of your trip, considering potential delays.

- Plan Rest Stops and Breaks: Incorporate frequent breaks and rest periods into your travel itinerary. Long journeys or extended periods of sitting can exacerbate MG symptoms. Plan for rest stops to stretch, relax, and recharge.

- Adapt Travel Plans to Your Abilities: Be realistic about your energy levels and physical capabilities. Modify travel plans and activities to suit your abilities, allowing for adequate rest and pacing activities throughout the trip.

- Stay Hydrated and Eat Well: Maintain hydration and nourishment during travel. Carry water and snacks to keep energy levels up. Stick to a balanced diet as much as possible to support overall well-being.

- Ensure Comfortable Accommodations: Choose accommodations that prioritize comfort and accessibility. Consider factors such as comfortable bedding, ease of movement within the room, and proximity to necessary facilities.

- Stay Mindful of Stress: Traveling can be stressful, and stress can trigger MG symptoms. Practice stress-reducing techniques such as deep breathing, mindfulness, or meditation to manage stress levels during travel.

Inspiring stories of individuals thriving with MG

Karen's Artistic Journey

Karen's life took an unexpected turn when she received the diagnosis of Myasthenia Gravis (MG) during her early twenties. Initially, the news left her feeling overwhelmed and uncertain about her future. Amidst the challenges of managing her symptoms, she discovered an unexpected outlet for her emotions – art.

At first, Karen tentatively picked up a paintbrush, dabbling in colors and shapes as a form of therapy. The act of painting provided her with a sense of calmness and control, an escape from the uncertainties that came with living with a chronic condition.

As she delved deeper into her newfound passion, Karen's art evolved. Her paintings began to reflect the emotional rollercoaster of living with MG – vibrant hues portrayed moments of hope and determination, while softer tones captured the challenges and vulnerabilities she faced.

Encouraged by friends and family, Karen showcased her artwork in a local community art fair. To her surprise, the response was overwhelming. Viewers were moved by the raw emotions captured in her paintings, and her artwork resonated with others experiencing similar health battles.

Buoyed by the positive reception, Karen started an art therapy group for individuals living with chronic illnesses. The sessions became a safe haven for participants to express themselves through art and share their stories. Karen's leadership and empathy helped foster a supportive community where individuals felt understood and inspired.

Her art journey took a new turn when a local gallery expressed interest in featuring her paintings. It was a significant milestone for Karen, who saw this as an opportunity to raise awareness about MG and the power of art in healing.

Karen's exhibit drew attention not just for its artistic brilliance but also for its underlying message. She used the platform to educate visitors about MG, sharing her story and those of others living with the condition. Her paintings became a catalyst for conversations, inspiring empathy and understanding among the attendees.

Through her art, Karen found purpose and meaning. It became a powerful tool not only for her self-expression but also for advocacy, creating a ripple effect that touched the lives of many. Karen's journey was a testament to the transformative power of creativity and resilience in the face of adversity.

Sophia's Parenting Journey

Sophia, a devoted mother, faced unexpected challenges when diagnosed with Myasthenia Gravis (MG) shortly after the birth of her first child. Coping with the demands of motherhood while managing the uncertainties of a chronic condition was daunting.

Initially, Sophia struggled to find a balance between caring for her newborn and prioritizing her health needs. Fatigue, muscle weakness, and fluctuating symptoms made daily caregiving tasks demanding. However, with unwavering support from her partner and family, Sophia gradually learned to adapt her parenting approach.

She discovered that pacing herself was essential. Sophia created a routine that accommodated her energy levels, strategically planning activities during her peak times and resting during moments of fatigue. She openly communicated with her partner about her limitations, fostering a supportive environment where they shared parenting responsibilities.

Sophia found creative ways to engage with her child, incorporating low-energy activities such as storytelling, cuddling, and interactive games that didn' t strain her physically. She sought assistance from family members and friends when needed, allowing for short breaks to recharge while ensuring her child received constant care and attention.

Education was a key aspect of Sophia's journey. She educated her family and friends about MG, explaining the condition and how it affected her ability to perform certain tasks. This understanding fostered a supportive network that provided help and encouragement whenever required.

Over time, Sophia's resilience and determination became an inspiration not only to her immediate family but also to other parents facing similar challenges. She joined online parenting communities, sharing her experiences and offering guidance to individuals navigating MG while raising children.

Sophia's parenting journey was characterized by adaptability, communication, and a steadfast commitment to both her health and her child's well-being. Despite the hurdles posed by MG, she found joy, fulfillment, and a profound sense of accomplishment in successfully navigating the intricacies of parenting while managing a chronic condition.

Chapter 9: Caregiver

Support and Resources

Understanding the Role of Caregivers in

MG Management

Caregivers play a pivotal role in the lives of individuals living with Myasthenia Gravis (MG), providing invaluable support, assistance, and care throughout the journey with the condition. Understanding the essential role of caregivers is crucial in comprehending their impact on MG management:

1. Providing Physical Support: Caregivers often assist individuals with MG in carrying out daily activities, including tasks that may become challenging due to muscle weakness or fatigue. This support ranges from

help with mobility and personal care to ensuring medication adherence and facilitating medical appointments.

2. Emotional Support and Encouragement: Caregivers offer emotional support by providing comfort, understanding, and encouragement. They play a significant role in boosting morale, being empathetic listeners, and providing reassurance during difficult moments.

3. Advocacy and Assistance in Communication: Caregivers often act as advocates for individuals with MG, ensuring their needs are understood and met within healthcare settings. They aid in effective communication with healthcare providers, helping convey symptoms, concerns, and treatment preferences.

4. Assistance in Daily Life Management: Caregivers assist in managing household responsibilities and organizing schedules to accommodate the needs of the individual with MG. They adapt routines and environments to ensure safety and comfort.

5. Monitoring and Observing Symptoms: Caregivers play a crucial role in observing and reporting changes in symptoms or health conditions to healthcare professionals. Their vigilance helps in timely interventions and adjustments to treatment plans.

6. Supporting Lifestyle Adjustments: Caregivers aid in adjusting lifestyle factors to better manage MG symptoms, including dietary modifications, stress reduction strategies, and encouraging regular exercise within the individual's capabilities.

7. Providing Respite and Self-care Opportunities: Caregivers also need support. Encouraging them to take breaks, offering respite care, and facilitating their self-care routines is crucial in preventing caregiver burnout and maintaining their well-being.

Self-care for Caregivers

In the realm of caregiver support and resources, focusing on self-care becomes paramount. Self-care is vital for caregivers managing the responsibilities and challenges of caring for someone with Myasthenia Gravis (MG). Encouraging caregivers to prioritize their own well-being is crucial in preventing burnout and maintaining their physical and mental health. Self-care strategies for caregivers involve setting boundaries, seeking support networks, and allocating time for personal activities that provide relaxation and rejuvenation. Engaging in hobbies, practicing mindfulness, exercising, seeking counseling or support groups, and ensuring adequate rest are essential components of self-care. By emphasizing self-care, caregivers can sustain their ability to provide effective and compassionate care while nurturing their own health and well-being.

Chapter 10: Conclusion

Summary of Key Takeaways

Throughout this comprehensive exploration of living with Myasthenia Gravis (MG), caregivers' roles, management strategies, and available resources, several key takeaways emerge:

1. Understanding Myasthenia Gravis (MG): MG is a chronic autoimmune neuromuscular disorder characterized by muscle weakness and fatigue. Knowledge about its symptoms, diagnosis, and impact on the neuromuscular system is crucial for effective management.

2. Caregivers' Vital Role: Caregivers play a pivotal role in supporting individuals living with MG. Their assistance, emotional support, and advocacy contribute significantly to managing the condition and enhancing the quality of life for those affected.

3. Management Strategies: Effective management of MG involves a multidisciplinary approach. This includes medications, treatments like thymectomy or plasma exchange, and lifestyle adjustments such as stress management, balanced nutrition, and adequate rest.

4. Challenges in Diagnosis: Diagnosing MG can be complex due to varied symptoms and the need for specific tests. Awareness of common symptoms and challenges in diagnosis assists in timely and accurate identification of MG.

5. Embracing Lifestyle Adjustments: Individuals with MG benefit from adapting their lifestyle to accommodate their energy levels and physical capabilities. Balancing physical activity, rest, stress reduction techniques, and healthy dietary choices are key components.

6. Support and Resources: Accessing available support networks, educational materials, caregiver resources, and patient advocacy organizations is vital for individuals and caregivers alike. These resources offer guidance, emotional support, and information essential in managing MG effectively.

7. Importance of Self-Care: Caregivers' self-care is crucial. Prioritizing personal well-being, seeking support, setting boundaries, and accessing respite care services are essential in preventing caregiver burnout and maintaining overall health.

8. Continuous Learning and Advocacy: Continuously seeking knowledge about MG, advocating for oneself or loved ones, and being proactive in accessing available resources are key elements in effectively managing the condition.

Final thoughts on thriving despite the

challenges of MG

Living with Myasthenia Gravis (MG) presents significant challenges, yet it's important to recognize that thriving is possible despite these obstacles. Thriving doesn't mean the absence of difficulties but rather finding strength, resilience, and hope amid the challenges posed by this chronic condition. The journey with MG is multifaceted, requiring a combination of medical management, lifestyle adjustments, support networks, and emotional resilience. While MG might impact daily life, it does not define the entirety of one's existence. The stories of resilience, the dedication of caregivers, and the relentless pursuit of knowledge and support are testaments to the human spirit's ability to overcome adversity. By embracing a multidisciplinary approach, seeking support, adapting lifestyle, and nurturing personal well-being, individuals and caregivers can foster a fulfilling life despite the complexities of MG. Remember, thriving is a journey, not a destination, and every step taken toward managing MG contributes to a life filled with resilience, purpose, and hope.

Glossary

1. Myasthenia Gravis (MG): A chronic autoimmune neuromuscular disorder characterized by muscle weakness and fatigue. It occurs when the immune system mistakenly attacks receptors on muscle cells, leading to impaired communication between nerves and muscles.

2. Acetylcholine: A neurotransmitter that transmits signals between nerve cells and muscle cells. In MG, antibodies can interfere with the acetylcholine receptors, leading to muscle weakness.

3. Thymus: A gland located in the chest behind the breastbone involved in the development of the immune system. It plays a role in some cases of MG, and surgical removal (thymectomy) can be a treatment option.

4. Thymectomy: Surgical removal of the thymus gland, sometimes performed in individuals with MG to

improve symptoms or reduce the need for immunosuppressive medications.

5. Autoimmune Disorder: A condition where the immune system mistakenly attacks the body's own cells and tissues, as seen in MG when antibodies attack the neuromuscular junction.

6. Neuromuscular Junction: The point of contact between a nerve cell and a muscle cell, where the transmission of signals occurs, allowing for muscle contraction. MG affects this junction, leading to muscle weakness.

7. Immunosuppressants: Medications that suppress the immune system's activity. They are often used in MG treatment to reduce the immune system's attack on the neuromuscular junction.

8. Pyridostigmine: A medication used in MG treatment that enhances the communication between nerves and muscles by inhibiting the breakdown of acetylcholine.

9. Plasmapheresis: A procedure that involves removing and replacing blood plasma. It is used in MG to remove harmful antibodies from the blood.

10. Intravenous Immunoglobulin (IVIG) Therapy: Treatment involving the infusion of antibodies collected from healthy donors. IVIG therapy is used in MG to modify the immune response and reduce symptoms.

11. Electromyography (EMG): A diagnostic test that measures the electrical activity in muscles. It helps in assessing muscle function and detecting abnormalities in MG.

12. Computed Tomography (CT) Scan: An imaging technique that uses X-rays to create detailed images of the body. CT scans are used to examine the thymus gland in individuals with MG.

13. Magnetic Resonance Imaging (MRI): An imaging technique that uses magnetic fields and radio waves to produce detailed images of the body's organs and tissues. It helps in evaluating the thymus and detecting abnormalities.

14. Dysphagia: Difficulty in swallowing, which can occur in individuals with MG due to weakness in the muscles involved in swallowing.

15. Diplopia: Double vision, a common symptom in MG caused by weakness in the eye muscles.

16. Dysarthria: Difficulty in speaking due to weakness in the muscles involved in speech production, commonly seen in MG.

17. Ptosis: Drooping of the eyelid, a characteristic symptom of MG caused by weakness in the muscles that lift the eyelids.

18. Dyspnea: Shortness of breath, which can occur in MG due to weakness in the muscles involved in respiration.

19. Fatigue: A prevalent symptom in MG characterized by extreme tiredness and weakness, often worsening with exertion.

20. Prednisone: A corticosteroid medication used in MG treatment to suppress the immune system's activity and reduce inflammation.

21. Azathioprine: An immunosuppressive medication used in MG treatment to prevent the immune system from attacking the neuromuscular junction.

22. Cyclosporine: An immunosuppressive drug used in MG treatment to control the immune system's response.

23. Tacrolimus: Another immunosuppressive medication used in MG treatment to prevent the immune system from attacking the neuromuscular junction.

24. Rituximab: A monoclonal antibody therapy used in MG treatment to target specific cells in the immune system and reduce their activity.

25. Methotrexate: An immunosuppressive medication used in MG treatment to suppress the immune system's response.

26. Azathioprine: An immunosuppressive medication used in MG treatment to prevent the immune system from attacking the neuromuscular junction.

27. Corticosteroids: A class of medications that suppress the immune system and reduce inflammation. They are commonly used in MG treatment.

28. Dysphonia: Difficulty in producing voice sounds due to muscle weakness, a symptom experienced by some individuals with MG.

29. Dysphagia: Difficulty swallowing, caused by weakened muscles in the throat, commonly seen in MG.

30. Dyspnea on Exertion: Shortness of breath experienced during physical activity due to muscle weakness, often seen in MG.

31. Fatigue Management: Various strategies, including pacing activities, resting, and energy conservation techniques, used to manage fatigue in MG.

32. Corticosteroid Tapering: Gradually reducing the dosage of corticosteroids to prevent adverse effects while maintaining MG control.

33. Comorbidities: Other health conditions that may coexist with MG, requiring additional management and care.

34. Modified Diet: Adjustments made to the diet to accommodate swallowing difficulties or to address specific nutritional needs in MG.

35. Mobility Aids: Assistive devices such as canes, walkers, or wheelchairs used to enhance mobility in individuals with muscle weakness due to MG.

36. Occupational Therapy: Therapy aimed at improving daily functional abilities and adaptation to MG-related limitations.

37. Dysarthria Therapy: Speech therapy aimed at improving speech clarity and strength in the muscles used for speech production.

38. Dysphagia Rehabilitation: Therapy focused on improving swallowing function and safety during eating and drinking.

39. Psychosocial Support: Emotional and psychological support provided by counselors,

therapists, or support groups to individuals and caregivers dealing with the impact of MG.

40. Care Plan: A personalized plan outlining the treatment, management strategies, and care requirements for individuals with MG.

41. Health-Related Quality of Life (HRQoL): A measure assessing the impact of health conditions on an individual's overall well-being and daily functioning in MG.

42. Neuromuscular Specialist: A healthcare professional specializing in the diagnosis and treatment of neuromuscular disorders, including MG.

43. Symptomatic Treatment: Treatment aimed at alleviating specific symptoms of MG without addressing the underlying cause.

44. Antibody Testing: Blood tests used to detect the presence of specific antibodies associated with MG.

45. Respiratory Support: Devices such as non-invasive ventilation or mechanical ventilation used to support

breathing in individuals with MG experiencing respiratory muscle weakness.

46. Symptom Flare-up: A sudden worsening of MG symptoms, often requiring adjustments in treatment or medical intervention.

47. Crisis Management: Strategies and plans in

 place to address severe MG exacerbations or myasthenic crises, which can be life-threatening.

48. Caregiver Fatigue: Physical or emotional exhaustion experienced by caregivers due to the demands of providing care for individuals with MG.

49. Caregiver Support Groups: Groups providing peer support, information, and resources specifically for caregivers of individuals with MG.

50. Adaptive Equipment: Tools or devices designed to assist individuals with MG in performing daily activities more easily and independently.

Appendices

Sample Meal Plans and Dietary

Guidelines

Proper nutrition plays a significant role in managing Myasthenia Gravis (MG) by supporting overall health and energy levels. While there's no one-size-fits-all diet for MG, certain dietary adjustments can help individuals cope with symptoms and optimize their nutritional intake. Below are some general dietary guidelines and sample meal plans that may be beneficial:

Dietary Guidelines for MG:

1. Balanced Diet: Aim for a well-balanced diet consisting of fruits, vegetables, whole grains, lean

protein sources, and healthy fats. Incorporate a variety of foods to ensure a diverse nutrient intake.

2. Frequent Meals: Opt for smaller, more frequent meals throughout the day to avoid fatigue associated with consuming larger meals. This approach helps maintain energy levels and minimizes muscle fatigue.

3. Hydration: Stay well-hydrated by drinking an adequate amount of water throughout the day. Dehydration can exacerbate MG symptoms, so it's essential to maintain proper hydration.

4. Protein Intake: Include adequate protein sources such as poultry, fish, tofu, legumes, and dairy products. Protein is essential for muscle strength and repair.

5. Limit Sugar and Refined Carbohydrates: Minimize the intake of sugary foods and refined carbohydrates as they can lead to energy fluctuations and fatigue.

6. Omega-3 Fatty Acids: Incorporate sources of omega-3 fatty acids such as fatty fish (salmon, mackerel), flaxseeds, chia seeds, and walnuts. Omega-

3s have anti-inflammatory properties and may benefit individuals with MG.

7. Calcium and Vitamin D: Ensure adequate intake of calcium and vitamin D through dairy products, fortified foods, leafy greens, and supplements if necessary. These nutrients support bone health, especially important for individuals on long-term corticosteroids.

Sample Meal Plan 1:

Breakfast:

- Greek yogurt with mixed berries and a sprinkle of nuts/seeds
- Whole grain toast with avocado or nut butter
- Herbal tea or water

Mid-Morning Snack:

- Apple slices with almond butter
- Water or herbal tea

Lunch:

- Grilled chicken or tofu salad with mixed greens, assorted vegetables, and olive oil vinaigrette
- Quinoa or brown rice on the side
- Water or herbal tea

Afternoon Snack:

- Carrot sticks with hummus
- Herbal tea or water

Dinner:

- Baked salmon or lentil stew
- Steamed vegetables (broccoli, carrots)
- Whole grain pasta or sweet potato
- Water or herbal tea

Evening Snack (if needed):

- Greek yogurt with honey or a small handful of nuts
- Herbal tea or water

Sample Meal Plan 2:

Breakfast:

- Scrambled eggs with spinach and tomatoes
- Whole grain toast
- Fresh fruit salad (berries, kiwi, or citrus fruits)
- Herbal tea or water

Mid-Morning Snack:

- Greek yogurt with a handful of granola
- Herbal tea or water

Lunch:

- Grilled chicken or chickpea salad with mixed greens, bell peppers, cucumber, and a light vinaigrette dressing
- Quinoa or brown rice on the side
- Water or herbal tea

Afternoon Snack:

- Sliced bell peppers with hummus
- Herbal tea or water

Dinner:

- Baked cod or baked tofu with roasted vegetables (zucchini, eggplant, bell peppers)
- Quinoa or wild rice
- Water or herbal tea

Evening Snack (if needed):

- Sliced apple with a small serving of cheese or a handful of nuts
- Herbal tea or water

Sample Meal Plan 3:

Breakfast:

- Overnight oats made with oats, almond milk, chia seeds, and mixed berries
- Whole grain toast with avocado
- Herbal tea or water

Mid-Morning Snack:

- Banana with a handful of nuts or seeds
- Herbal tea or water

Lunch:

- Turkey or tempeh wrap with whole grain tortilla, lettuce, tomatoes, and hummus
- Mixed fruit salad
- Water or herbal tea

Afternoon Snack:

- Celery sticks with peanut butter
- Herbal tea or water

Dinner:

- Grilled shrimp or tofu stir-fry with assorted vegetables (bell peppers, broccoli, snap peas) in a light sauce
- Brown rice or cauliflower rice
- Water or herbal tea

Evening Snack (if needed):

- Cottage cheese with pineapple or a small portion of popcorn
- Herbal tea or water

Breathing Exercises for Myasthenia Gravis

Breathing exercises can help improve respiratory muscle strength and manage breathlessness in individuals with Myasthenia Gravis (MG). Perform these exercises in a comfortable, seated position with proper posture:

1. Diaphragmatic Breathing (Abdominal Breathing):

- Sit comfortably in a chair with your feet flat on the floor and your back straight.
- Place one hand on your chest and the other on your abdomen, just below the rib cage.
- Inhale slowly and deeply through your nose, allowing your abdomen to rise while keeping your chest relatively still.
- Exhale slowly through pursed lips, gently drawing your abdomen inward.
- Repeat this breathing pattern for several breaths, aiming for a slow and controlled rhythm.

2. Segmental Breathing:

- Sit comfortably and place your hands on the sides of your rib cage.
- Inhale slowly and deeply, directing the breath into the lower part of your lungs, allowing the ribs to expand outward.
- Hold the breath for a few seconds, then exhale slowly, gently contracting the abdominal muscles to push the air out.
- Next, focus on breathing into the middle part of your lungs, expanding the rib cage sideways.
- Hold briefly, then exhale slowly, allowing the ribs to contract back to the starting position.
- Finally, focus on breathing into the upper part of your lungs, expanding the chest and raising the rib cage.
- Exhale slowly, allowing the chest to relax.
- Repeat this segmented breathing, gradually progressing from lower to middle to upper lung segments.

3. Pursed Lip Breathing:

- Inhale slowly through your nose for a count of two or three seconds.

- Purse your lips as if you're going to whistle or blow out a candle.
- Exhale slowly and gently through pursed lips for a count of four to six seconds.
- This technique helps maintain open airways and prevents rapid exhalation.

4. Deep Breathing with Arm Movement:

- Sit comfortably with your back straight.
- Inhale deeply through your nose, raising both arms overhead, reaching toward the ceiling.
- Exhale slowly through pursed lips, lowering your arms back to your sides.
- Repeat this deep breathing while raising and lowering your arms several times, focusing on a relaxed and controlled breathing pattern.

Perform these breathing exercises daily or as recommended by your healthcare provider. These exercises aim to improve lung capacity, promote relaxation, and enhance respiratory muscle function in individuals managing MG.

Range of Motion Exercise Routine for

Myasthenia Gravis

Note: Perform each exercise smoothly and slowly, avoiding any jerky movements. If any exercise causes pain or discomfort, stop immediately.

1. Neck Flexion and Extension:

- Sit or stand in a comfortable position with the spine straight.
- Gently lower the chin towards the chest, feeling a stretch at the back of the neck. Hold for 5-10 seconds.
- Slowly tilt the head backward, looking upward, and feeling a stretch at the front of the neck. Hold for 5-10 seconds.
- Repeat this flexion and extension movement 5-8 times.

2. Shoulder Rolls:

- Relax your shoulders and gently roll them forward in a circular motion.

- Perform 5-8 forward shoulder rolls.
- Then, reverse the motion and roll the shoulders backward in a circular motion for 5-8 repetitions.

3. Arm Circles:

- Extend your arms to the sides at shoulder height.
- Slowly rotate your arms in small circles clockwise, making the circles slightly larger with each rotation.
- Perform 5-8 clockwise arm circles.
- Reverse the direction and perform 5-8 counterclockwise arm circles.

4. Wrist Flexion and Extension:

- Extend your arms in front of you at shoulder level, palms facing downward.
- Gently bend your wrists upward, aiming to bring the fingers toward the ceiling.
- Hold the stretch for 5-10 seconds, feeling the stretch in the front of the wrists.
- Then, reverse the movement by bending the wrists downward, aiming to point the fingers toward the floor.
- Hold the stretch for 5-10 seconds, feeling the stretch in the back of the wrists.

- Repeat wrist flexion and extension 5-8 times.

5. Ankle Alphabet:

- Sit in a chair with one foot lifted off the ground or lie down comfortably with one leg extended.
- Rotate your ankle in a circular motion, tracing the letters of the alphabet with your big toe.
- Complete the alphabet in both clockwise and counterclockwise directions.
- Repeat with the other foot/leg.

Strengthening Exercises Routine for

Myasthenia Gravis:

Warm-up:
Begin with a gentle warm-up to prepare the muscles for exercise. Perform light cardiovascular activity such as walking or cycling for 5-10 minutes.

1. Seated Leg Extension:
- Sit comfortably in a chair with your back straight and feet flat on the floor.
- Slowly extend one leg out in front of you, keeping the knee straight but not locked.
- Hold the extended position for 5-10 seconds.
- Slowly lower the leg back to the starting position.
- Repeat 10-15 times for each leg, alternating sides.

2. Seated Leg Press:
- Sit in a chair with your feet flat on the floor.
- Press your foot against an immovable object (like a wall or heavy object) in front of you, engaging the muscles in your thighs.
- Hold the press for 5-10 seconds, then release.

- Repeat this press with both legs, aiming for 10-15 repetitions for each leg.

3. Seated Row:
- Sit on the edge of a chair or a stability ball with your back straight and feet flat on the floor.
- Hold a resistance band or tubing securely in front of you with both hands.
- Pull the band towards your torso, bending your elbows and squeezing your shoulder blades together.
- Slowly release back to the starting position.
- Aim for 10-15 repetitions.

4. Bicep Curls with Resistance Band:
- Sit comfortably with a straight back, holding a resistance band in both hands with palms facing up.
- Curl your hands towards your shoulders, keeping your elbows close to your sides.
- Slowly lower your hands back to the starting position.
- Perform 10-15 repetitions.

5. Chest Press with Resistance Band:
- Sit tall on a chair or stability ball, holding the resistance band at chest level.

- Push the band forward, extending your arms but keeping a slight bend in your elbows.
- Return to the starting position.
- Aim for 10-15 repetitions.

Cool Down:
Finish your routine with a gentle cool-down. Perform some light stretching exercises focusing on the muscles worked during the routine. Hold each stretch for 15-30 seconds without bouncing.

Important Tips:
- Start with low resistance and gradually increase as tolerated.
- Focus on controlled movements and proper form rather than speed or quantity.
- Take breaks as needed and listen to your body. Stop immediately if you experience pain or excessive fatigue.
- Perform these exercises 2-3 times per week, allowing for rest days in between sessions.

Balance and Coordination Exercises

Routine

Note: Perform these exercises at a pace comfortable for you, and always have a stable support nearby (like a chair or countertop) for safety if needed.

1. One-Leg Stand:

- Stand near a stable surface (such as a countertop or chair) for support if necessary.
- Lift one foot off the ground slightly while maintaining balance.
- Aim to hold this position for 10-15 seconds.
- Switch legs and repeat on the other side.
- Perform 3-5 repetitions on each leg, gradually increasing the duration as your balance improves.

2. Tandem Walk:

- Find a clear space to walk a straight line.

- Stand with one foot directly in front of the other (heel-to-toe) in a straight line.
- Walk forward, placing one foot directly in front of the other with each step.
- Focus on maintaining balance and walking steadily along the line.
- Perform this exercise for about 20-30 steps, ensuring proper posture and steady movement.

3. Ball Toss and Catch:

- Sit comfortably on a stable surface or stand with a partner at a comfortable distance.
- Toss a soft ball or a lightweight object back and forth, focusing on catching and throwing with accuracy.
- Start with gentle tosses and gradually increase the speed or distance as you feel more comfortable.
- Aim for 10-15 tosses back and forth.

4. Eyes Closed Balance:

- Stand in a comfortable position with feet shoulder-width apart and arms by your sides.
- Close your eyes gently and focus on maintaining your balance without visual cues.

- Hold this position for about 10-15 seconds or as long as comfortable.
- Gradually increase the duration as your balance improves.

5. Single Leg Toe Touch:

- Stand near a stable surface for support if needed.
- Lift one leg slightly off the ground while balancing on the other leg.
- Slowly bend at the waist and reach down to touch the toes of the balancing leg with the opposite hand.
- Return to the starting position with control.
- Perform 8-10 repetitions on each leg.

6. Heel-to-Toe Walk:

- Stand upright with one foot in front of the other, placing the heel of one foot directly in front of the toes of the other.
- Walk in a straight line, placing the heel of the front foot in front of the toes of the back foot with each step.
- Focus on maintaining proper balance and coordination as you take each step.

- Perform this exercise for about 20-30 steps in one direction and then return.

Posture Improvement Exercises Routine:

Note: Perform each exercise slowly and gently. Stop immediately if you experience any discomfort or increased weakness.

1. Seated Spinal Stretch:

- Sit on a stable chair with feet flat on the floor and hands resting on thighs.
- Inhale, lengthen the spine, and gently twist your upper body to the right, placing the left hand on the right knee.
- Exhale as you twist a little deeper, feeling a gentle stretch in your spine.
- Hold for 10-15 seconds, then slowly return to the center.
- Repeat on the other side, twisting gently to the left. Aim for 3 repetitions on each side.

2. Chin Tucks:

- Sit or stand with your back straight and shoulders relaxed.

- Gently draw your chin inward without tilting your head up or down.
- Hold the position for 5-10 seconds while maintaining a straight gaze forward.
- Relax and return to the starting position. Aim for 10-15 repetitions.

3. Shoulder Blade Squeeze:

- Sit or stand comfortably with arms by your sides.
- Squeeze your shoulder blades together, as if you're trying to hold a pencil between them.
- Hold the squeeze for 5-10 seconds while maintaining normal breathing.
- Relax and repeat for 10-15 repetitions.

4. Wall Angels:

- Stand with your back against a wall, feet shoulder-width apart, and arms bent at 90 degrees with palms facing forward.
- Slowly slide your arms up the wall, maintaining contact between your elbows, wrists, and the wall.
- Move your arms upward until fully extended overhead (without forcing if it causes discomfort).

- Hold for a couple of seconds, then slowly return to the starting position. Aim for 10-15 repetitions.

5. Pelvic Tilts:

- Sit on a chair with your feet flat on the floor and hands resting on your thighs.
- Gently tilt your pelvis backward, flattening the lower back against the chair.
- Hold the position for 5-10 seconds, feeling the engagement in your lower abdominal muscles.
- Relax and return to the starting position. Repeat 10-15 times.

6. Cat-Cow Stretch:

- Start on your hands and knees with a neutral spine (tabletop position).
- Inhale, arch your back, and lift your head and tailbone upwards (cow position).
- Exhale, round your spine, tuck your chin to your chest, and tuck your tailbone under (cat position).
- Flow smoothly between the cow and cat positions for 5-10 repetitions, coordinating with your breath.

Low-Impact Aerobic Exercise Routine for

MG:

Please note: Consult a healthcare professional before starting any exercise routine, and perform these exercises at a pace comfortable for you. Stop immediately if you experience any pain or discomfort.

1. Warm-up (5-10 minutes):

- Start with gentle warm-up activities such as walking in place, marching, or easy arm swings to gradually increase heart rate and loosen muscles.
- Perform light stretching focusing on major muscle groups, including arms, legs, back, and shoulders, holding each stretch for about 15-30 seconds.

2. Aerobic Activity (15-30 minutes):

Choose one or a combination of low-impact aerobic activities:

a. Walking:

- Walk at a comfortable pace indoors or outdoors. Start with 5-10 minutes if you're a beginner, gradually increasing the duration as tolerated.
- Use proper footwear and maintain good posture while walking.

b. Stationary Cycling:

- Use a stationary bike at a comfortable resistance level. Pedal at a steady pace for 10-15 minutes, gradually increasing the duration over time.
- Maintain proper posture and adjust the seat to a comfortable height.

c. Swimming or Water Aerobics:

- Perform water-based exercises in a pool under supervision if available. Engage in activities like water walking, gentle swimming, or water aerobics.
- Take advantage of the water's buoyancy to reduce impact on muscles and joints.

d. Elliptical Trainer or Recumbent Bike:

- Use an elliptical trainer or a recumbent bike with adjustable resistance. Start with 5-10 minutes and gradually increase the duration as tolerated.
- Maintain a comfortable pace and avoid overexertion.

3. Cool Down (5-10 minutes):

- Slow down the pace of the activity, gradually reducing intensity.
- Perform gentle stretching exercises targeting major muscle groups, holding each stretch for about 15-30 seconds.
- Practice deep breathing or relaxation techniques to help bring heart rate and breathing back to normal.

4. Hydration and Rest:

- Drink water to stay hydrated before, during, and after the exercise routine.
- Listen to your body and rest if needed. It's important to avoid excessive fatigue.

5. Monitoring:

- Monitor how you feel during and after the exercise routine. Pay attention to any unusual fatigue, weakness, or discomfort.
- Adjust the duration and intensity of the exercises according to your comfort level and any recommendations from your healthcare provider.

6. Frequency:

- Aim for at least three sessions per week, gradually increasing the frequency as tolerated.

Modified Yoga Routine for Myasthenia

Gravis:

1. Breathing Exercises (Pranayama):
   - Sit comfortably in a chair or on a yoga mat with proper support.
   - Practice deep breathing exercises, focusing on diaphragmatic breathing. Inhale deeply through the nose, expanding the abdomen, and exhale slowly through the mouth.

2. Gentle Warm-up:
   - Begin with gentle joint movements and neck stretches to release tension. Rotate the neck slowly, gently stretch the arms, wrists, and ankles.

3. Seated Mountain Pose (Tadasana):
   - Sit tall with feet flat on the floor, spine aligned, and shoulders relaxed.
   - Inhale and reach arms overhead, stretching upward. Exhale and release arms down.
   - Repeat for several breaths, focusing on elongating the spine.

4. Seated Forward Fold (Paschimottanasana Variation):
   - Sit with legs extended in front, back straight.
   - Inhale and lengthen the spine. Exhale, hinge at the hips, and fold forward, reaching towards the feet or shins.
   - Hold the stretch for a few breaths, maintaining a gentle stretch without straining.

5. Seated Twist (Ardha Matsyendrasana Variation):
   - Sit tall with legs extended or bent, spine lengthened.
   - Inhale and lift through the crown of the head. Exhale, twist gently to the right, placing the left hand on the right knee and the right hand behind.
   - Hold the twist for a few breaths, then switch sides.

6. Supported Warrior Pose (Virabhadrasana Variation):
   - Sit or stand with support nearby.
   - Place one foot forward, bend the front knee slightly, and keep the back leg straight.
   - Raise arms gently to shoulder height or use support if needed, feeling a stretch in the legs and torso.
   - Hold the pose for a few breaths, then switch legs.

7. Relaxation (Savasana):

  - Lie down comfortably on a yoga mat or in a chair, allowing the body to relax completely.

  - Close the eyes and focus on deep, relaxed breathing for a few minutes.

Modified Pilates Routine for Myasthenia

Gravis:

1. Breathing and Centering:
  - Begin in a comfortable seated or lying position, focusing on diaphragmatic breathing to center and connect with the body.

2. Pelvic Tilts (Pelvic Curl):
  - Lie on the back with knees bent, feet flat on the floor.
  - Inhale, engage the abdominal muscles, and tilt the pelvis upward, lifting the hips slightly. Exhale and lower back down.
  - Repeat the movement, focusing on pelvic stability and controlled movements.

3. Leg Slides (Leg Circles Modification):
  - Lie on the back with knees bent.
  - Slowly slide one leg along the floor, extending it gently and then returning to the starting position.

- Perform a few slides on each leg, keeping movements controlled and within a comfortable range.

4. Modified Hundreds:
   - Lie on the back with knees bent, arms by the sides.
   - Inhale, lift the head and shoulders off the mat, and extend the arms alongside the body.
   - Exhale and lower back down, repeating the movement in a controlled manner.

5. Seated or Supported Spine Stretch Forward:
   - Sit tall with legs extended or slightly bent.
   - Inhale and lengthen the spine. Exhale, hinge at the hips, and reach forward, keeping the back flat.
   - Use support if needed and focus on stretching the back muscles gently.

6. Breathing and Relaxation:
   - End the routine with deep breathing and relaxation techniques, allowing the body to unwind and relax completely.

These exercise guidelines and sample meal plans are meant to provide general insights into a balanced diet and lifestyle suitable for individuals managing MG. However, it's essential to consult with a healthcare professional or a registered dietitian to create a personalized nutrition plan tailored to individual needs, taking into account any specific dietary restrictions, medications, or symptoms related to MG.

Worksheets for Symptom Tracking and

Medication Management

Managing Myasthenia Gravis (MG) involves keeping track of symptoms, medication schedules, and their effects on daily life. Utilizing worksheets for symptom tracking and medication management can help individuals and healthcare providers gain insights into the condition's patterns and better tailor treatment strategies. Below are sample worksheets that can be used or customized to suit individual needs:

1. Symptom Tracking Worksheet:

Date: _____

Symptoms Experienced:

- Fatigue levels (Low/Medium/High)
- Muscle weakness (Mild/Moderate/Severe)
- Difficulty swallowing (Yes/No)
- Double vision (Yes/No)
- Shortness of breath (Yes/No)

- Speech difficulties (Yes/No)
- Other symptoms: _____

Factors Influencing Symptoms:

- Stress levels (Low/Medium/High)
- Sleep quality (Poor/Fair/Good)
- Physical activity (Low/Medium/High)
- Medication changes (Yes/No)
- Dietary changes (Yes/No)
- Other factors: _____

Notes/Comments:

Note: Use this worksheet to track daily symptoms, their severity, and potential influencing factors. Discuss findings with your healthcare provider during appointments.

2. Medication Management Log:

Date: _____

Medication Name: _____

Dosage/Strength: _____

Frequency: _____

Time Taken: _____

Effectiveness Rating: (On a scale of 1-10)

- Symptom relief
- Side effects
- Overall impact on daily life

Notes/Comments:

Note: Use this log to record medication details, dosage, time taken, effectiveness, and any side effects experienced. Discuss this log during healthcare appointments for medication adjustments or modifications.

3. MG Flare-Up Action Plan:

In collaboration with your healthcare provider, create an action plan detailing steps to take during MG symptom flare-ups or exacerbations. Include emergency contacts, medication dosage adjustments, and when to seek immediate medical assistance.

These worksheets are designed to assist individuals in monitoring MG symptoms, tracking medication usage, and preparing for potential flare-ups. They can serve as useful tools in enhancing communication with healthcare providers, aiding in personalized treatment plans, and managing MG more effectively on a day-to-day basis. Customize these worksheets as needed and consult healthcare professionals for guidance on using them effectively.

Printed in Great Britain
by Amazon

49027945R00086